117 Health Tips

A quick guide for a healthy life

Professor Norman Ratcliffe

Cranmore Publications

Illustrated by Hannah Michael

A catalogue record for this book is available from the British Library

ISBN: 978-1-907962-08-0

Published by Cranmore Publications

Reading, England

www.cranmorepublications.co.uk

For Teri

Contents

About the Author

- **Professor Norman Ratcliffe** is a founder member of a team that recently discovered a new antibiotic potentially capable of curing MRSA and *Clostridium difficile*. This work was presented to Prince Phillip at St. James's Palace, London and was the subject of major media attention in the UK on ITV News and in many leading newspapers, including the Wall Street Journal, around the World. He is a Fellow of the Royal Society of Medicine and has previously run a "Health Alert" blood-testing company. He has published over 200 books and research papers on immunology, cancer invasion, influenza, tropical diseases and MRSA. He played squash for Wales, ran the London Marathon at the age of 50 and works-out regularly in the gym.

- **Professor Ratcliffe** retired recently after 25 years as a University Research Professor. He decided to finally complete his main book on health "It's Your Life" after 5 years work in order to help the many people who are confused about health and fitness issues and who have constantly been asking his advice.

Introduction

The purpose of this book is to provide helpful tips which will help you to maintain your health, fitness and strength throughout your life.

I hope that the tips are of great value to you. You will find that many of the tips have associated illustrations aimed at bringing the advice to life and making it more memorable.

After reading this book, you may require more detailed information concerning the tips. Indeed, you will notice that many tips contain chapter references for "It's Your Life". This is the name of my comprehensive book on health; it is a treasure trove of valuable information concerning health and fitness. You can find more information about "It's Your Life" at the end of this book.

117 Health Tips

Tip 1

Never skip breakfast, as it is the most important meal of the day and will help to control your weight by reducing snacking.

Tip 2

A healthy breakfast could include a low sugar cereal (see "It's Your Life") or oatmeal plus skimmed/semi-skimmed milk, wholemeal bread and/or fresh fruit.

Tip 3

Get rid of children's breakfast cereals containing high sugar levels e.g. "Coco Pops", "Frosties" and some muesli. Replace these with low sugar cereals such as "Weetabix" and "Shredded Wheat".

Tip 4

If you are late in the morning then always find time to nibble on a piece of bread or fruit to replace your usual breakfast.

Tip 5

Kick those fried breakfasts into touch! Gradually reduce the number that you have each week.

Tip 6

Eat Oatmeal Porridge for the perfect breakfast food as it contains low fat and salt and reduces cholesterol levels.

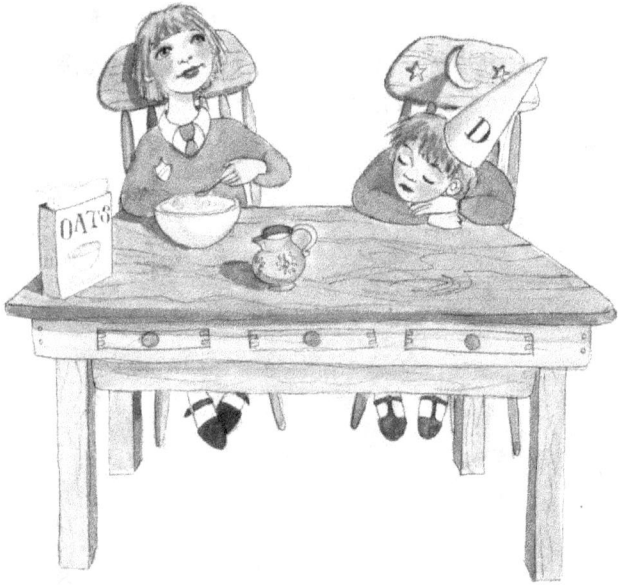

Tip 7

Eating breakfast results in higher concentration and better school work in children as well as increased energy levels and improved behaviour and well-being.

Tip 8

Get rid of white bread today! It is chemically dyed
white and devoid of any beneficial nutrients or fibre.
Even fortified white lacks fibre and some nutrients.

Showing wholemeal and white loaves and the possible advantages and disadvantages of eating each type of bread

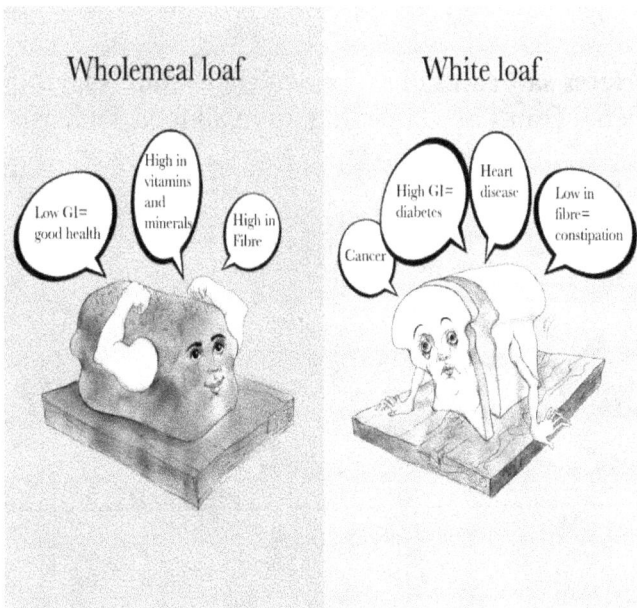

Tip 9

Excess salt can kill so for adults the limit is no more than 6 grams of salt per day from all food sources.

Shows that excess salt raises blood pressure and causes strokes and heart disease

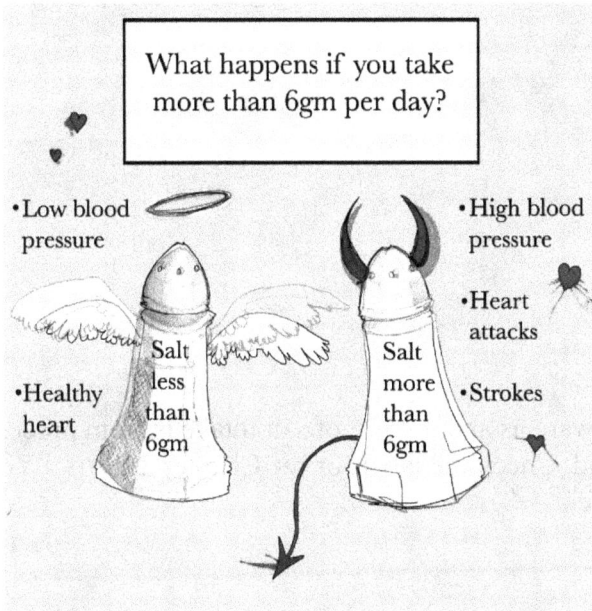

What happens if you take more than 6gm per day?

• Low blood pressure

• Healthy heart

Salt less than 6gm

• High blood pressure

• Heart attacks

Salt more than 6gm

• Strokes

Tip 10

Beware some bread, such as Hovis Extra Thick, Square Cut White, which contains 1 gram of salt per slice!

Tip 11

Beware as about 75 % of salt intake is from processed food. Check the labels or see Chapter 2 in "It's Your Life".

Tip 12

Confused by salt content on food packaging? Remember, 2 grams of "sodium" = 2 x 2.5 = 5 grams of salt.

Tip 13

Children less than 14 yr old need less than the 6 grams salt per day recommended for adults. Thus, 7-10 yr =5 grams, 4-6 yr = 3 grams, 1-3 yr = 2 grams and less than 1 yr = 0.5-1 gram per day.

Tip 14

To protect against bowel cancer eat red meat only 1-2 times per week. Red meat includes beef, lamb, bacon, gammon and pork.

Tip 15

Avoid processed meats such as hotdogs, sausages, and pepperoni as they are even worse than red meat for association with cancer of the bowel.

Tip 16

To reduce your intake of harmful saturated fats, replace whole milk with skimmed (24 times less saturated fat than whole milk) or semi-skimmed milk, especially in coffee and cereals.

Tip 17

DON'T BE GULLIBLE. NEVER take notice of publicity on health and diet from TV "celebrities". They know little except how to extract your money and usually fail to follow their own advice!

Tip 18

Men should always use the ketchup freely even in restaurants! Cooked tomato products such as ketchup and tomato juice may protect men against prostate cancer.

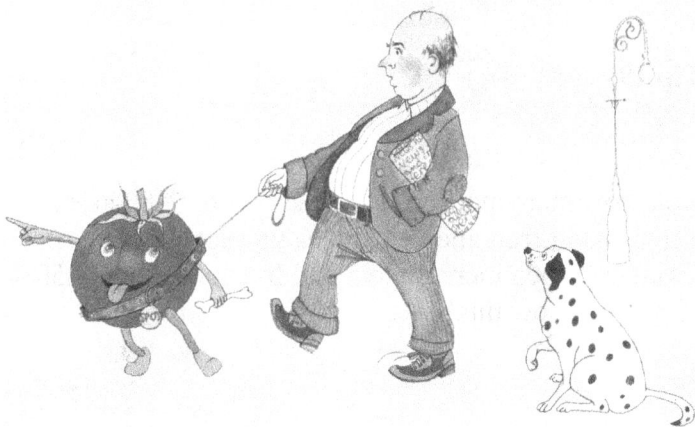

Tip 19

Note how many portions (i.e. one portion = 80 grams = 3 ounces) of fruit and vegetables you eat each day. If less than 5 then increase to 5 and live longer. Only 50% of people know this!!!

Shows the benefits of eating at least 5 portions of fruit and vegetables per day

Fruit and Vegetables

Reduce risk of strokes, heart disease and cancer	Low in fat and calories and help in weight control

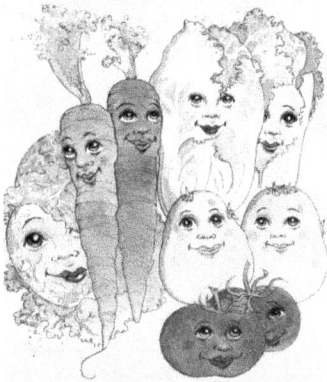

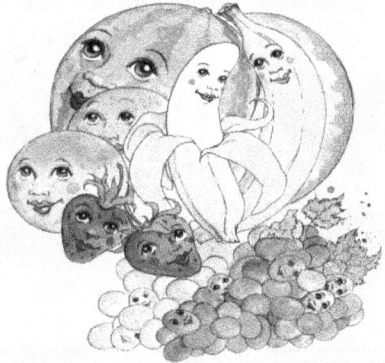

Tip 20

Are you eating a healthy diet with a balance of carbohydrates, proteins, fruit and vegetables at every meal? Eating healthily means that you can still have cakes, sweets, crisps and junk occasionally but only as a reward.

Shows the main groups of foods described opposite. The size of each slice represents the proportion of the diet that should contain that food group. Hence the smallest slice contains sweets, biscuits, cakes etc. Note that meat and dairy products have been combined into one slice

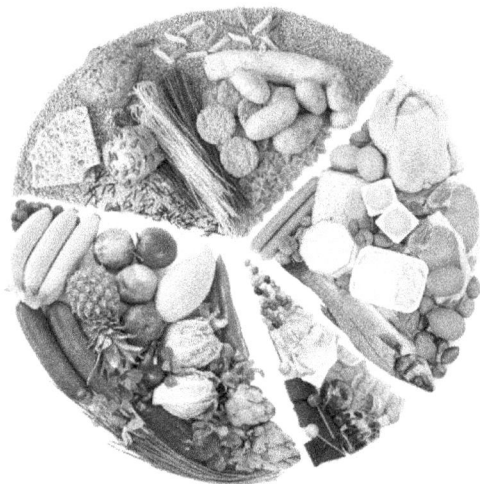

Tip 21

Junk food rich in fat and sugar is addictive so make GRADUAL changes to improve your diet.

Tip 22

IN THE UK, drink tap water as there is little evidence that bottled water is purer. Bottled water is often stored for 1-2 years before drinking allowing chemical leaching from the plastic!

Tip 23

Drink plenty of water throughout the day to detoxify the body and to prevent constipation and fatigue. Usually 6-8 glasses is advised but dark yellow and strong-smelling urine indicates dehydration.

Tip 24

To avoid weight gain with age either reduce food intake or increase amount of exercise.

Tip 25

Are you more than 40 yr old and gaining weight?
Probably your physical activity has reduced. LIST
REASONS for loss of activity and then you will
understand your weight gain. Read "It's Your Life" for
details.

Shows some of the reasons for declines in physical activity

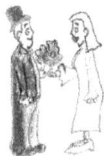

Marriage

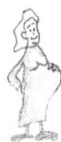

Pregnancy

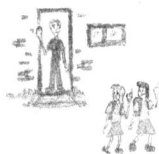

Children grown up

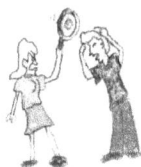

Divorce

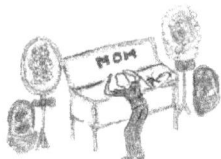

Bereavement

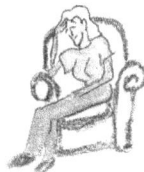

Depression

Tip 26

Always remember that weight gain will occur when **"calories eaten exceed calories used by the body".**

Tip 27

Women are more likely to gain weight with age due to lower metabolism resulting from a lower muscular mass than men.

Tip 28

BEWARE, do not reduce your food intake drastically at the same time as you increase your exercise or you will greatly stimulate your appetite.

Tip 29

REMEMBER to change your lifestyle slowly so that your new diet and exercise regimens become a natural part of everyday living.

Tip 30

For details at a glance of calories, fat, salt, fibre and sugar of over 300 common foods see Chapter 2, Table 1 of "It's Your Life".

Tip 31

BEGINNING TODAY, reduce processed foods and pre-prepared meals in your diet like pies, pizzas, quiches, pastas, curries, burgers etc, as these are full of calories, saturated fats, salt, sugar and additives. Slowly begin to re-introduce home cooked meals, salads etc and regain control over what you eat.

Tip 32

Beware buying sandwiches, as they are usually full of calories, saturated fats and salt. Make your own!!

Tip 33

Beware soft drinks such as Colas, flavored waters, fizzy drinks, Fanta, lemonade and many **fruit juice drinks** which often have high levels of additives, added sugar and very little fruit.

Tip 34

Only drink fruit juices labeled as 100% natural fruit and not those labeled "cranberry, orange, apple **fruit drink**" which will contain a mixture of additives.

Tip 35

Understand fats in food. Good fats are monounsaturated and polyunsaturated found in vegetable oils and oily fish. Bad fats are saturated fats and trans fatty acids found in full fat dairy products, fatty meat products, cakes and biscuits.

Tip 36

Avoid white bread like the plague!!!!! People who eat white bread may suffer higher rates of heart disease, some cancers and diabetes.

Tip 37

Include enough high fibre foods (made with wholemeal flour, as well as in many fruits and vegetables) in your diet to prevent constipation and other gut problems including cancer.

Tip 38

Reducing the saturated and trans fatty acids in your diet will decrease your risk of heart disease. Find out more in Chapter 3 of "It's Your Life".

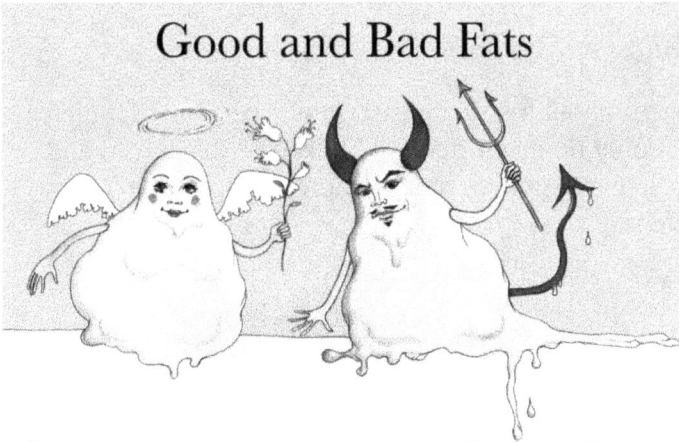

Good and Bad Fats

Monosaturates and
Polyunsaturates

Saturated and
Trans fatty acids

Tip 39

Forget about trendy diets such as Atkins and GI diets. Not only do they often fail but can be dangerous and difficult to stick to. Read Chapters 1-3 in "It's Your Life".

Tip 40

86 % of people going on diets never actually lose weight. For dietary and weight control advice see Chapters 1-2 in "It's Your Life".

Showing some of the high fat foods originally recommended by Atkins

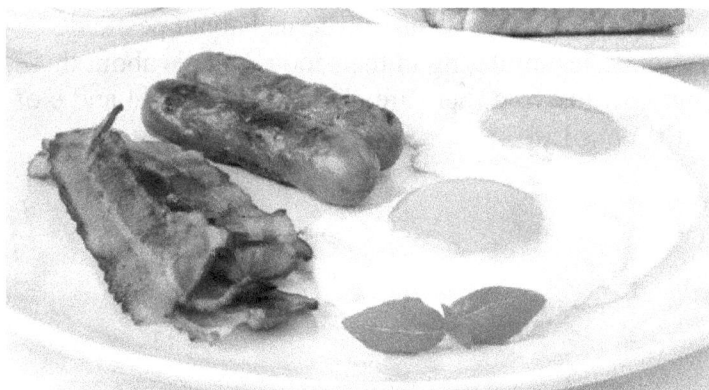

Tip 41

Nearly 60% of people are concerned about pesticide residues accumulating in their food. Details about these and how to avoid them are given in Chapters 4 and 6 of "It's Your Life".

Showing the origin of chemical residues in our food

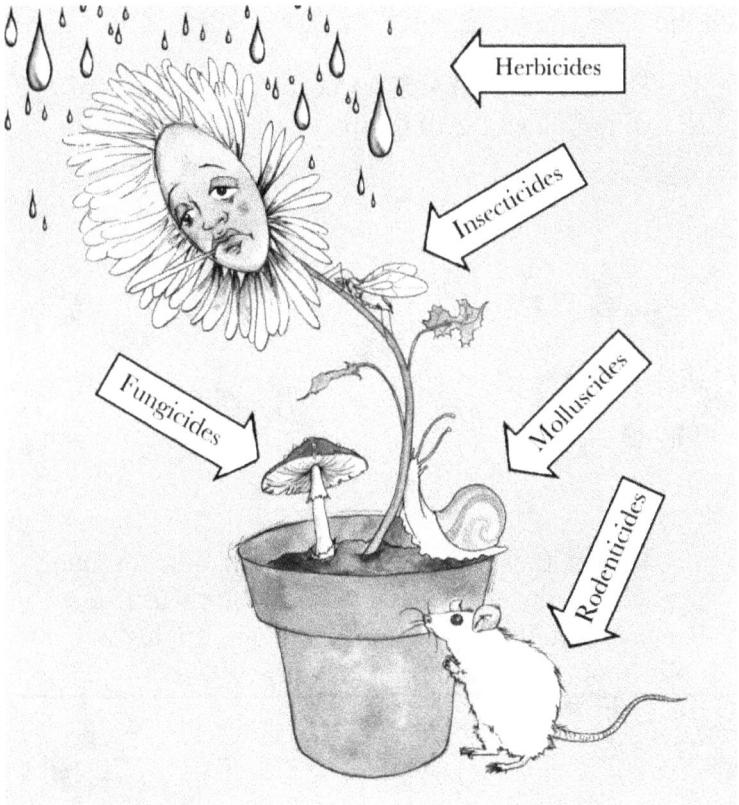

Tip 42

The best and worst foods for pesticide contents are
shown in Tables 1-3 of Chapter 4 of "It's Your Life".

Tip 43

The lowest rates of pesticide contamination are found
in peeled fruits and vegetables, such as citrus fruits,
bananas, mangoes, pineapples, melons, apples and
onions, potatoes, turnips, peas etc.

Tip 44

The highest rates of pesticide contamination are found in unpeeled "soft" fruits, such as grapes, strawberries, apricots, raspberries, cherries, plums, peaches and unpeeled apples and pears as well as unpeeled vegetables including salads, green beans, peppers, tomatoes etc.

Tip 45

Cereals and cereal products, such as wheat flour, rye, bran, oats, rice, bread, cereal bars, and breakfast cereals, have high rates of pesticide contamination. Buy organic if possible.

Tip 46

To reduce your intake of pesticide residues, use peeled fruit and vegetables or wash unpeeled items for 5 min in cold water.

Tip 47

Organic foods have very low pesticide residue levels but are expensive. Concentrate on buying organic potatoes, bread, cereals and cereal products, such as porridge oats, which are available at reasonable prices.

Tip 48

There are over 300 food additives approved for use but
their intake can be reduced by reading Chapter 5 of
"It's Your Life".

Tip 49

Most "diet", "light" or "zero" products contain artificial
sweeteners. High-powered advertising campaigns are
trying to promote these chemical mixes to gullible
children and adults.

Tip 50

Children are particularly vulnerable to the side effects of food additives taken in excessively in soft drinks and sweets. Safety concerns about the extensive use of food additives are detailed in Chapter 5 of "It's Your Life".

Showing a bowl of sweets and the E numbers of colourants used as additives

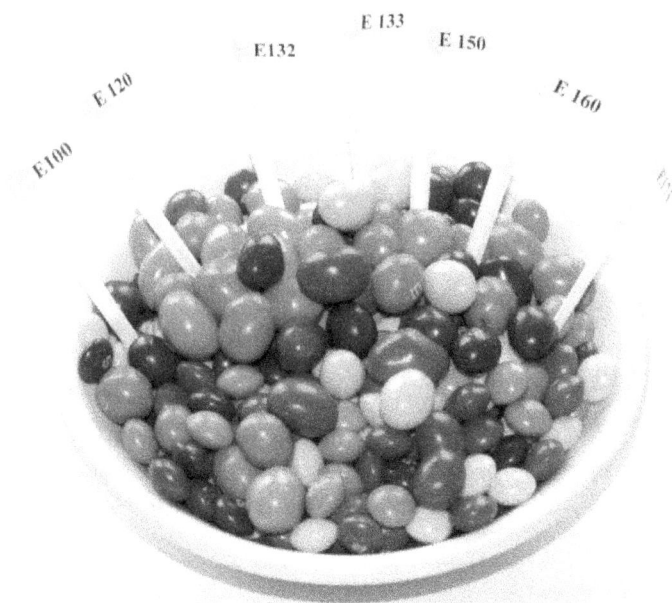

Tip 51

Reduce the intake of food additives by reducing processed foods in the diet.

Tip 52

Although some manufacturers are removing colorant additives from many sweets and medicines, these still contain sulphite preservatives, which can aggravate allergies.

Tip 53

Many cosmetics, beauty and hair products may also contain chemical preservatives. Check yours out.

Tip 54

Foods containing artificial sweeteners are often junk foods with low nutritional values.

Tip 55

Avoid "Sweet'N Low" (in that attractive little pink packet), which is a mixture of acesulfame and aspartame, and is widely used as a sweetener in coffee shops.

Tip 56

Beware monosodium glutamate, present in many foods to enhance flavor. The Co-op and other supermarkets have removed it from their own brands and from baby foods.

Tip 57

Avoid sulphite and benzoate preservatives as well as artificial colorants to reduce allergic responses, particularly in children. See, Chapters 5 and 6 of "It's Your Life".

Tip 58

Dilute squash/soft drinks for young (less than 4.5 yr) children to reduce excessive cyclamate sweetener intake.

Tip 59

Chemicals are taken in from many sources in the environment. These chemicals form the "BODY BURDEN" and may interact to cause disease. Learn how to reduce this "COCKTAIL EFFECT" in Chapter 6 of "It's Your Life".

Shows the origin of the many chemicals that we are exposed to and which form a cocktail in the body

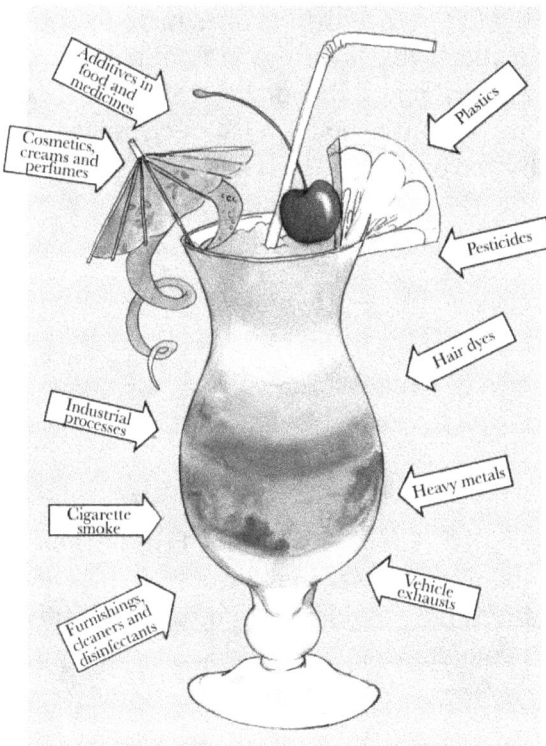

Tip 60

Beware the terms "healthy" and "natural" found on labels. To check the flavorings present in drink/food look at the label and if it contains real fruit extract then it is natural but if it contains a list of chemicals it is artificially flavored.

Tip 61

AVOID TOXIC CHEMICALS IN THE YOUNG. Understand that foetuses in the womb, babies and rapidly developing children will be more sensitive to chemical contaminants than adults.

Tip 62

Toxic chemicals can be passed to the unborn child in the mother's milk and be harmful to the foetus at levels regarded as "safe" for adult women.

Tip 63

Evidence from wildlife studies indicates how harmful environmental chemical contaminants can be in the body.

Tip 64

Reduce your body burden of contaminant chemicals, (i.e. detox) if you are trying for a baby.

Tip 65

Protect your family from contaminant chemicals in household products. Check Chapter 6 of "It's Your Life" for the sources of the most toxic chemicals in the body.

Tip 66

Are you one of the 43 million people in the UK who need vitamin and mineral supplements??? Find out in Chapters 7 and 8 of "It's Your Life".

Tip 67

End the confusion! Organic fruit and vegetables definitely contain significantly higher levels of antioxidants than conventionally-farmed produce.

Tip 68

If you can't afford organic food then eat locally grown, fresh food to optimize vitamin and mineral content. Failing this, frozen foods have limited nutrient loss and fewer chemical additives.

Tip 69

Vitamins may interact with medicines. BEFORE taking vitamin or mineral supplements check with your doctor that they do not interact with any medicines you are taking.

Tip 70

Vitamin supplements required vary at different stages of life. Avoid confusion and check out in Chapter 8 of "It's Your Life" which supplements you need.

Tip 71

It is difficult to obtain adequate requirements of vitamin D from the diet alone, as exposure of the skin to sunlight is required for the body to make this vitamin.

Tip 72

If you are one of the 13% of men and 15% of women who eat at least 5 fruit or vegetables per day and have a well balanced diet then you may **only** require a vitamin D supplement.

Tip 73

In the UK, 60 % of adults are vitamin D deficient and this is particularly a problem during spring and winter when it may reach 90%.

Tip 74

Vitamin D supplements are ESSENTIAL for people who cover the skin, are elderly, never go outside or live in Northern climates with limited sunshine.

Tip 75

In order to make sufficient vitamin D, exposure of face, legs, arms etc to the sun for 10-15 minutes per day, 2-3 times per week without sunscreen (but with no burning), is recommended.

Tip 76

Cod liver oil should be avoided by smokers, pregnant women and elderly people as it contains high vitamin A levels, which may damage the bones or cause cancer in smokers.

Tip 77

Multivitamins are safe as long as you take just **one per day** and take the appropriate one for your age group. Avoid those with more than the recommended daily allowance of vitamin A.

Tip 78

It is not generally recommended that people with a balanced diet, in the 19-59 yr age group, take high doses of antioxidants such as vitamins C, E and selenium.

Tip 79

Calcium supplementation may be required if you avoid dairy produce due to lactose intolerance or adopt a vegan lifestyle.

Tip 80

People taking glucosamine supplements for joint pain should take glucosamine **hydrochloride** and not glucosamine **sulphate** if they have high blood pressure.

Tip 81

Women intending to conceive or who are pregnant are recommended to take 400 micrograms of **folic acid (vitamin B9)** per day as a supplement to reduce the chances of spina bifida.

Tip 82

70% of teenage girls may be vitamin D deficient so that supplementation may be highly beneficial.

Tip 83

Taking a multivitamin supplement is highly beneficial for teens and associated with healthier lifestyles.

Tip 84

Elderly people are prime candidates for vitamin supplementation to help avoid the downward spiral of aging. See Chapter 8 of "It's Your Life" for details.

Tip 85

In elderly people deprived of sunlight, a vitamin D dose of 700-800 IU (17.5-20 micrograms) per day is recommended to reduce falls and fractures.

Tip 86

Recent work has shown that when heavy drinking is associated with smoking then the age of onset of Alzheimer's disease can be **6-7 years earlier**.

Tip 87

Low levels of vitamin D, due to low intake or lack of exposure to the sun, may increase the risk of developing diabetes.

Tip 88

Vitamin D deficiency has now been shown to be higher in obese people than in the normal population.

Tip 89

Endurance athletes, such as regular marathon runners, tri-athletes, cyclists etc, may obtain protection against the very high levels of radicals generated by these sports by taking antioxidant supplements.

Tip 90

To aid in their absorption, vitamins should generally be taken with a meal or snack.

Tip 91

Do not take your vitamins with hot drinks or drinks containing caffeine which is present in tea, coffee, colas etc. Caffeine inhibits the absorption of some vitamins and minerals.

Tip 92

There are liquid vitamins for people who find pills or capsules difficult to swallow.

Tip 93

Remember, regular exercise will help to protect you against heart disease, strokes, diabetes, cancer and even mental problems.

Tip 94

If adopting a new healthy eating and regular exercise lifestyle then **begin slowly** and gradually introduce your new diet and exercise regimens.

Tip 95

Consult your doctor if you have not taken regular exercise for a long time and wish to embark on a new strenuous exercise regimen.

Tip 96

Just walking 2 or more miles per day will reduce cancer and heart disease 2-3 fold in people over 50 years old.

Tip 97

New to the gym? Pick a user-friendly gym not filled with steroid freaks, aerobic goddesses and unhelpful instructors playing with their computers. YMCA and local authority gyms may be optimal for you.

Avoid gyms full of enormous steroid freaks as you will be intimidated and probably receive scant attention from the instructors

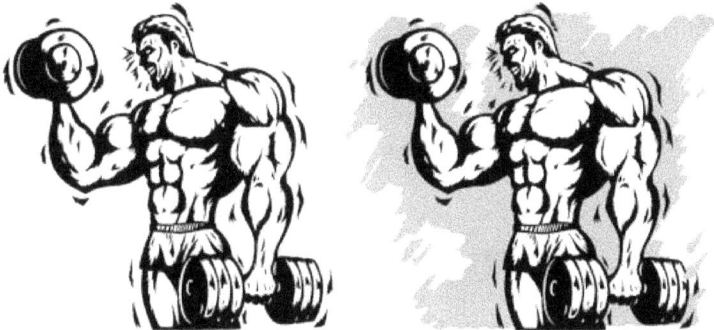

Tip 98

The gym is not suitable for everybody so find the type of exercise to which your temperament and body are best suited. See Chapters 10 and 11 of "It's Your Life" for help.

Tip 99

Never be frightened to ask for help with equipment or with your technique from fellow gym users or the instructors.

Tip 100

Beginning the gym for the first time? Make sure that you obtain a detailed exercise programme from the instructors (your induction) and that this is regularly updated with no extra charge.

Tip 101

Try and find someone to train with you as **"Gym Buddies"** are worth their weight in gold and often can correct your technique and provide much-needed motivation.

Tip 102

To boost your performance and minimize injury, always warm up on the treadmill, rower etc in the gym for 10 min and then stretch before beginning any exercise.

Tip 103

Overweight and embarking on exercise? Reduce your weight before running on hard surfaces outside or on the treadmill in the gym as these **may damage your joints**. Begin by using the rower, cross-trainer or static bike in the gym or walk or cycle outside.

Tip 104

Spin classes using static bikes are a fantastic way to shed weight and get fit.

Tip 105

How long ago did you last exercise for 20-30 min so that your pulse rate increased and talking was difficult??? Ensure at least 3 such exercise sessions per week.

Tip 106

Talking for long periods in the gym with friends is self-delusional and will inhibit progress.

Tip 107

With weights, sets of 15-20 repetitions with low weight will tone the body whilst sets of 6-10 with high weights will increase muscular size and strength.

Tip 108

Discover how many calories your type of exercise/sport uses per hour in Chapter 11 of "It's Your Life".

Tip 109

Discover the effects on cardiovascular function and joint damage of your type of exercise/sport in Chapter 11 of "It's Your Life".

Tip 110

Overweight and still snacking? Find out how long you need to walk, swim, cycle or run to burn the calories in that chocolate or cake! See Chapter 11 of "It's Your Life".

Tip 111

Muscle wasting begins at 40 yr old and accelerates through the 50s, 60s and 70s until frailty and inability to live independently results. Avoid frailty and begin a routine of weight-bearing exercises, for example, with dumbbells, press-ups etc.

Tip 112

If you need to snack then eat healthy snacks – see Chapter 11 of "It's Your Life".

Tip 113

Always ensure that you drink sufficient water before, during and after exercise. Dehydration will weaken your performance.

Tip 114

You are never too old, even in your 80-90s, to begin some form of weight-bearing exercise to avoid muscle wasting and frailty.

Showing the author's elderly neighbor using dumbbells to strengthen arms and shoulders

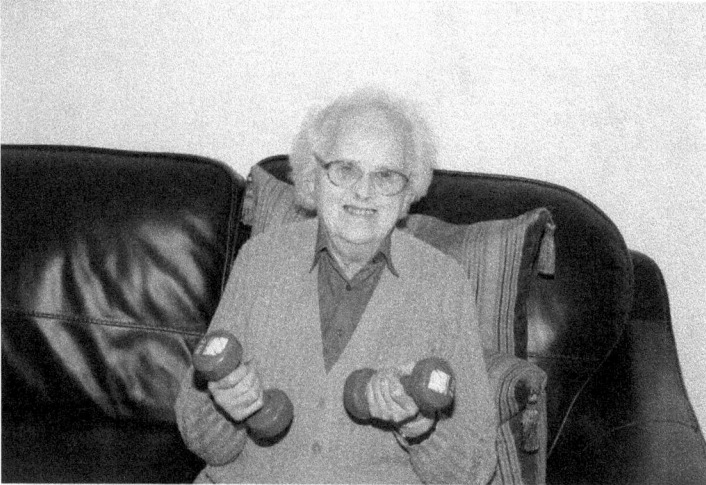

Tip 115

Diet and exercise requirements change at different times of life. Discover which exercise/sports are optimal for your age group by reading Chapter 11 of "It's Your Life".

Tip 116

Swimming is an excellent exercise for the heart and lungs but is of limited use as a weight-bearing exercise to ward off muscle wasting and frailty.

Tip 117

Demanding job and young family and no time for regular exercise? Build an exercise programme into your household tasks; see Chapter 11 of "It's Your Life".

It's Your Life

This section of the book provides some information about Professor Norman Ratcliffe's comprehensive book on health: *It's Your Life: End the confusion from inconsistent health advice.*

The main aim of "IT'S YOUR LIFE" is to end the confusion resulting from the huge outpouring of conflicting health advice appearing in the media almost daily. For example: Should we drink tap or bottled water? Is it necessary to buy solely organic foods? Are we being poisoned by pesticides and food additives? Are vitamin supplements really necessary and which ones should we take? Do we have to exercise 5 times per week? All advice offered is based on the analysis of existing scientific evidence and does not result from any alliance to a Government Organisation, an Alternative Health or

Lifestyle Charity, or a Pharmaceutical Company. This book does not profess to tell you how to live to be a 100 years old but it does show you, SIMPLY, how to maintain health, fitness, strength, energy and a feeling of well-being throughout your life and into your later years.

"IT'S YOUR LIFE" also aims to change our present concepts and prejudices that often compartmentalise people into certain categories at specific ages. Why is it that even well-meaning advertisements often portray 40+ people as unattractive and generally 50+ people as old, toothless, inactive and one step from the nursing home? The problem is that people are exposed to so much of this stereotyping that they subconsciously believe the hype and begin to live their lives accordingly.

"IT'S YOUR LIFE" IS A UNIQUE CONTRIBUTION SINCE:

- **It is for people of all different ages,** aiming to optimise health and fitness and maximise an active and independent lifestyle throughout life. It is not a part of the recent deluge of health and diet books or videos produced by B-class "celebrities" but has been written by a biomedical scientist of international repute.

- You will not find in most books **high impact illustrations** emphasising important points in the text. For example, the cover illustrates the present-day frustration and confusion of the average consumer exposed to contradictory health and dietary advice.

- You will not find in most books on diet and exercise clear summaries of **basic facts for adopting a new health plan.** Thus, for the many people with busy lives who may hate reading health books Chapter 1

("Food, The Basic Diet"),Chapter 9 ("Exercise, Basic In-troduction") and other Chapters are designed for rapid reference, often to specific age-groups of people.

- You will also not find in most other books descriptions of how many aspects of **diet and exercise change at different times of life** (Chapter 1) as well as reasons for weight gain as we age and advice as how to avoid this (Chapter 2, "Help! What Am I Eating?").

- You will also not find in most other books **extensive tables for rapid identification of foods containing high levels of calories, saturated fats, salt and sugar** (Chapter 2). Thus, information on over 300 different food groups can be extracted at a glance without the necessity of reading minute and confusing Supermarket Food Labels.

- You will also not find in most books **not only clearly tabulated facts** about **"The Good, The Bad And The Ugly Fats", and "Fibre"** but also appraisals of the Atkins and GI **"Fad Diets"** (Chapter 3).

- You will also not find in other books **details of the rates of pesticide contamination of fruit, vegetables and other types of food** using easily interpreted tables (Chapter 4). A summary table is also included, for attaching to the refrigerator door or notice board, to identify **the least chemically polluted foods.**

- You will also not find in other books **a list of organic foods that are the most important to buy** (Chapter 4) and an explanation why, in these financially challenged times, it is **unnecessary** to eat just organic foods.

- You will also not find in many other books **details of the potential impact on food safety of Food Additives, Preservatives and Colourants** (Chapter 5) together with consideration of the **total chemical loading** of the body from all sources (Chapter 6, "The Cocktail Effect"). Possible interactions of chemicals accumulated from pesticides and additives in food, and from cosmetics and household sources, are also discussed, and advice is given on **reducing the uptake of chemicals from the environment**.

- You will also not find in other books an understanding of the **"Vitamin Dilemma"** as **"To Take Or Not To Take, That Is The Question"** (Chapters 7 and 8) facing most people following conflicting advice in the media. Clear scientific analysis of the latest research shows that people require different supplements at different stages in their lives. **Supplement recommendations are made for each stage from pregnancy to old age.**

- You will also not find in most other books **an understanding of the "To Gym Or Not To Gym-That Is The Question" dilemma faced by many people beginning to exercise for the first time** (Chapter 9). It introduces the basics and benefits of regular exercise, describes how to begin training in the gym, and provides an outline exercise programme (Chapter 10).

- You will also not find in most other books **details of "Alternative Types Of Exercise For Gym–Haters"** (Chapter 11), with different sports and activities described together with the calories used and **a table of the time taken with different sports to burn off highly calorific snacks.** Uniquely, the effects of each type of exercise are presented in terms of joint damage and cardiovascular function, and **advice on exercising at different ages** is also included.

- In summary, **"IT'S YOUR LIFE",** presents the best advice available for optimising health and fitness in a manner designed to enlighten and engage the non-expert reader.

*Other books in the **117 Tips** range:*

117 Tips for a Spiritual Life

Simon Saint   (2011)

www.ingramcontent.com/pod-product-compliance
Lightning Source LLC
Chambersburg PA
CBHW050545280326
41933CB00011B/1731